MEATLESS MEAL

RECIPE BOOK

Johanna Earthly Ramos

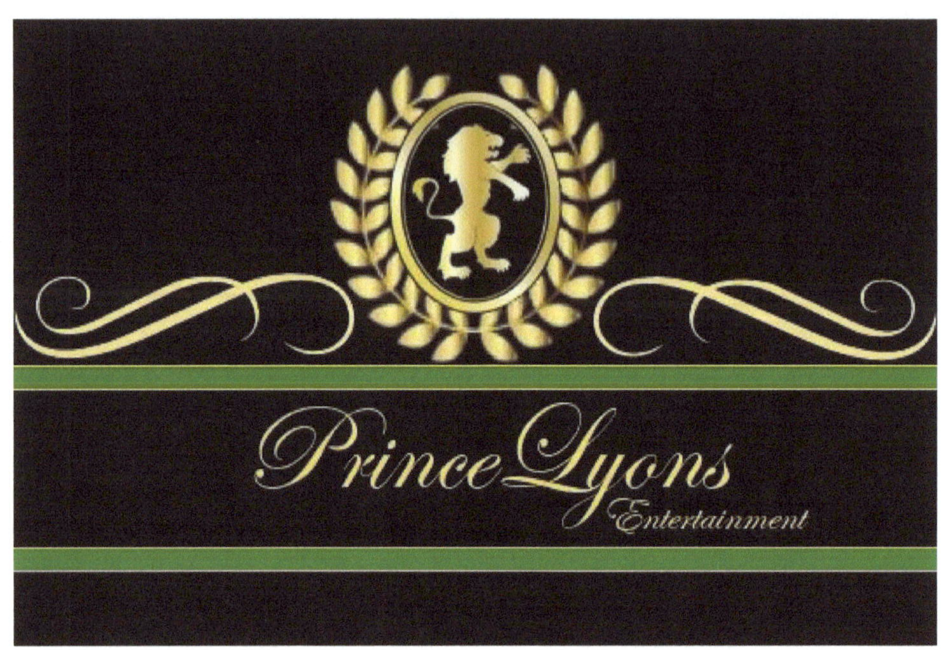

EARTHLY BODIES PRESENTS: MEATLESS MEAL RECIPE BOOK

Copyright ©2018

PrinceLyons Entertainment

www.princelyonsentertainment.com

Library of Congress Catalog Card Number:

ISBN-13: 978-1726276801

ISBN-10: 1726276805

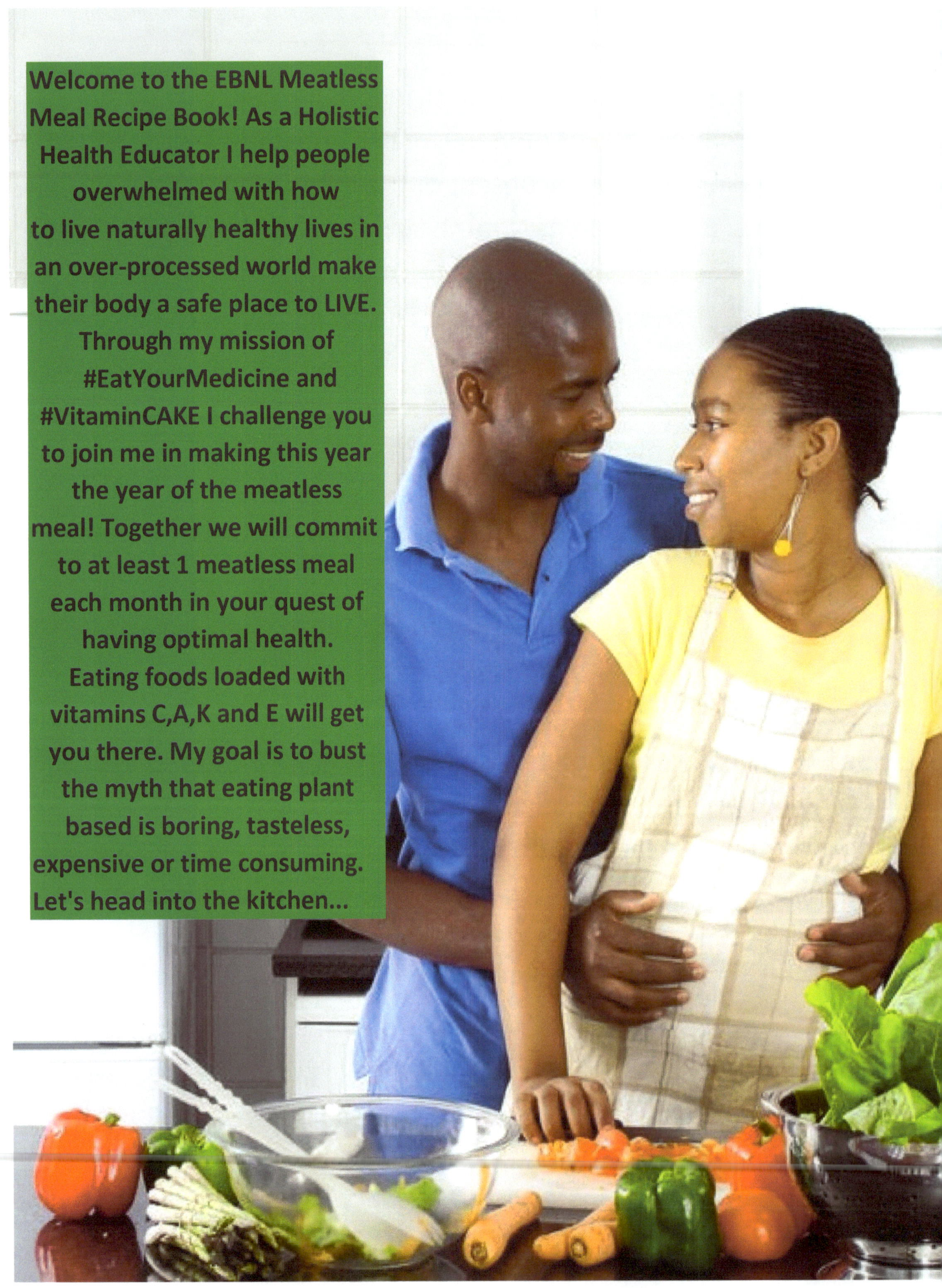

Welcome to the EBNL Meatless Meal Recipe Book! As a Holistic Health Educator I help people overwhelmed with how to live naturally healthy lives in an over-processed world make their body a safe place to LIVE. Through my mission of #EatYourMedicine and #VitaminCAKE I challenge you to join me in making this year the year of the meatless meal! Together we will commit to at least 1 meatless meal each month in your quest of having optimal health. Eating foods loaded with vitamins C,A,K and E will get you there. My goal is to bust the myth that eating plant based is boring, tasteless, expensive or time consuming. Let's head into the kitchen...

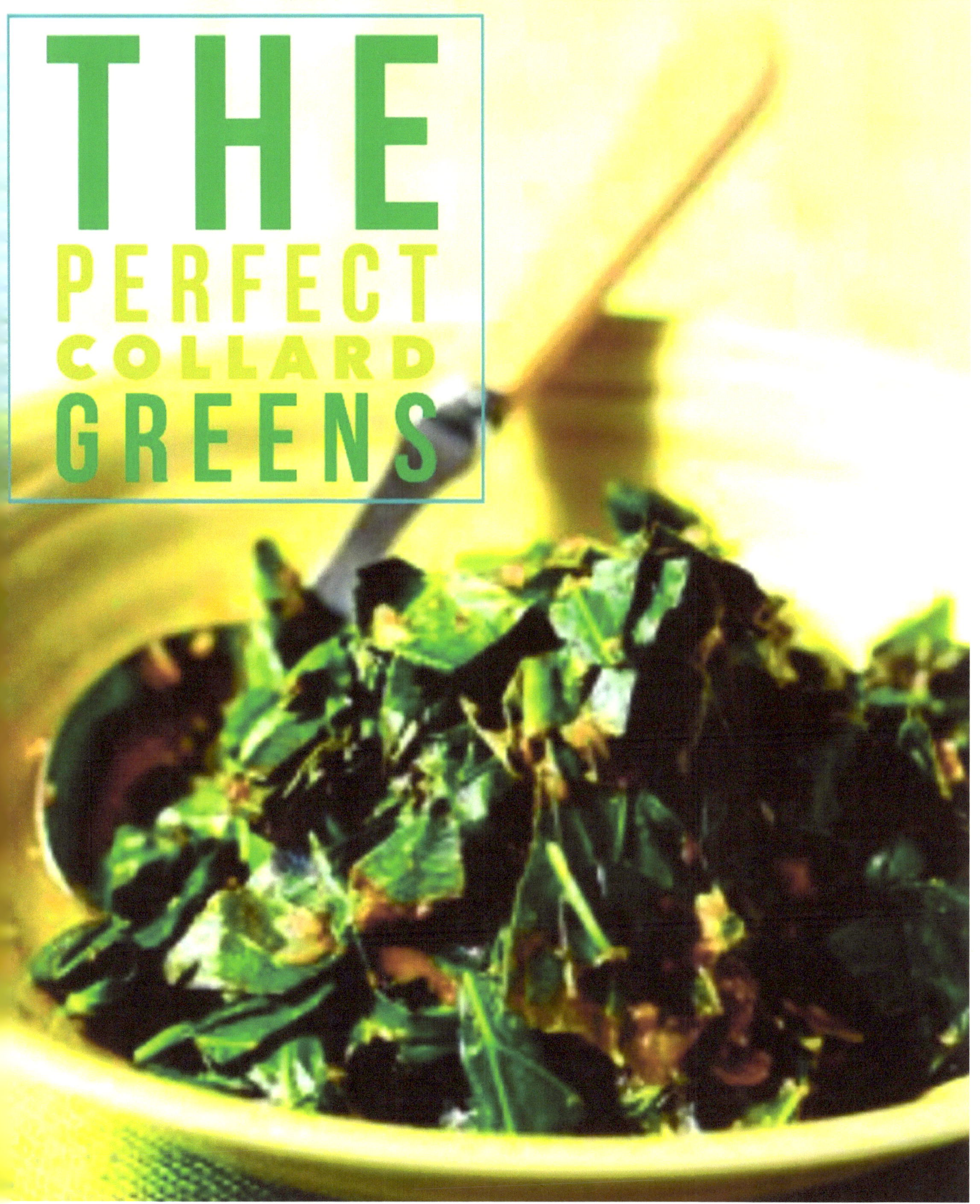

THE
PERFECT
COLLARD
GREENS

Collard greens are delicious AND nutritious! They are loaded with all the vitamin CAKE as well as calcium, protein and fiber. So, with all that magic why are we literally cooking our greens to death by leaving them on the stove for hours and adding unnecessary animal protein for flavor? Raise your right hand and repeat after me: I will no longer cook my greens to death because I want to join the mission to #EatYourMedicine. Pair The Perfect Collard Greens with the Skillet Sweet Potatoes

1 large bunch of collard greens sliced and chopped thin

3 Tbsp olive oil

1 cup diced onion

1 Tbsp minced garlic

1 Tbsp crushed red pepper flakes

1 Tbsp brown sugar

1/2 cup vegetable broth

1 Tbsp Himalayan pink salt

1 Tbsp black pepper

Add the oil to a large pan over medium-high heat. Add onions, garlic and crushed red pepper flakes. Cook until slightly caramelized (2-3 minutes) Place greens in the pan and toss to wilt a bit.

Add the brown sugar and vegetable broth. Toss together Turn the heat down and cover. Cook until liquid is evaporated, and greens look glazed. Toss occasionally for 10 minutes Season with salt and pepper.

Serve.

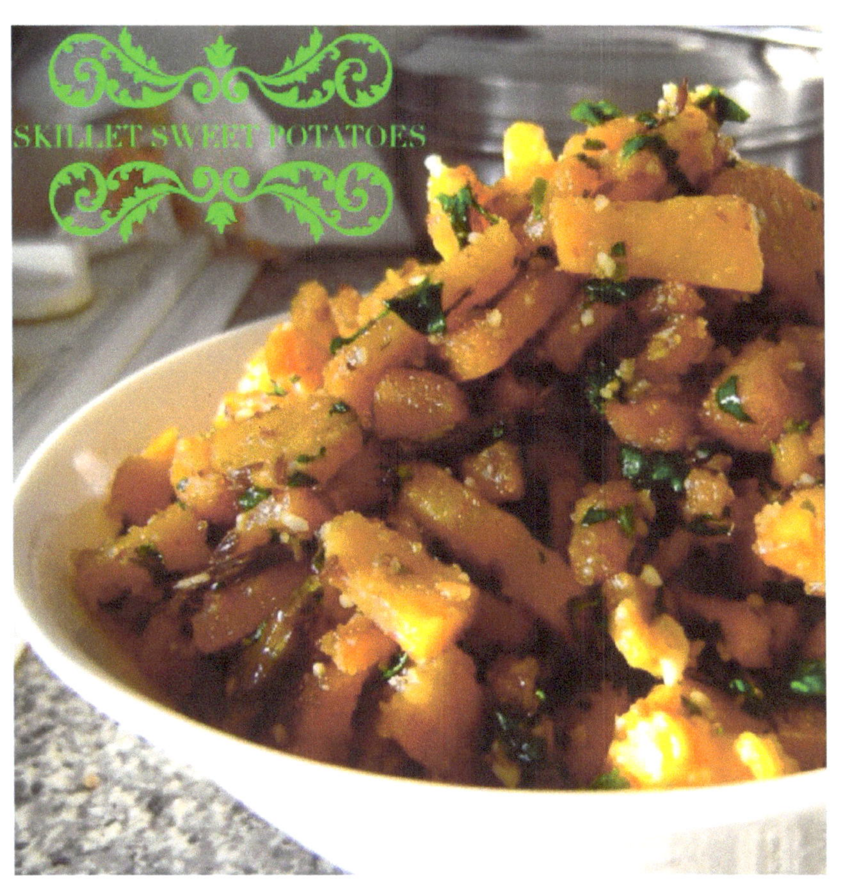

Enjoy these yummy Skillet Sweet Potatoes with The Perfect Collard Greens.

3 medium sweet potatoes
2 cloves garlic, minced
1 tsp Himalayan Pink Salt
2 TBSP fresh parsley, chopped
1/2 tsp ground cinnamon
1 TBSP coconut oil

Peel and cube sweet potatoes.
Heat up a skillet with oil, add the potatoes and stir.
Cook for about 15 minutes or until tender.
Stir often, making sure not to burn them.
Add minced garlic, salt, cinnamon and parsley.
Stir repeatedly and cook for another 4 minutes.
Stir often and try not to burn the garlic.
Enjoy when done!

*As an alternative you can roast these too. Preheat oven to 425F and just add all the ingredients to a roasting pan. Stir and bake for about 25-35 minutes depending on oven type and the size of your sweet potato cubes.

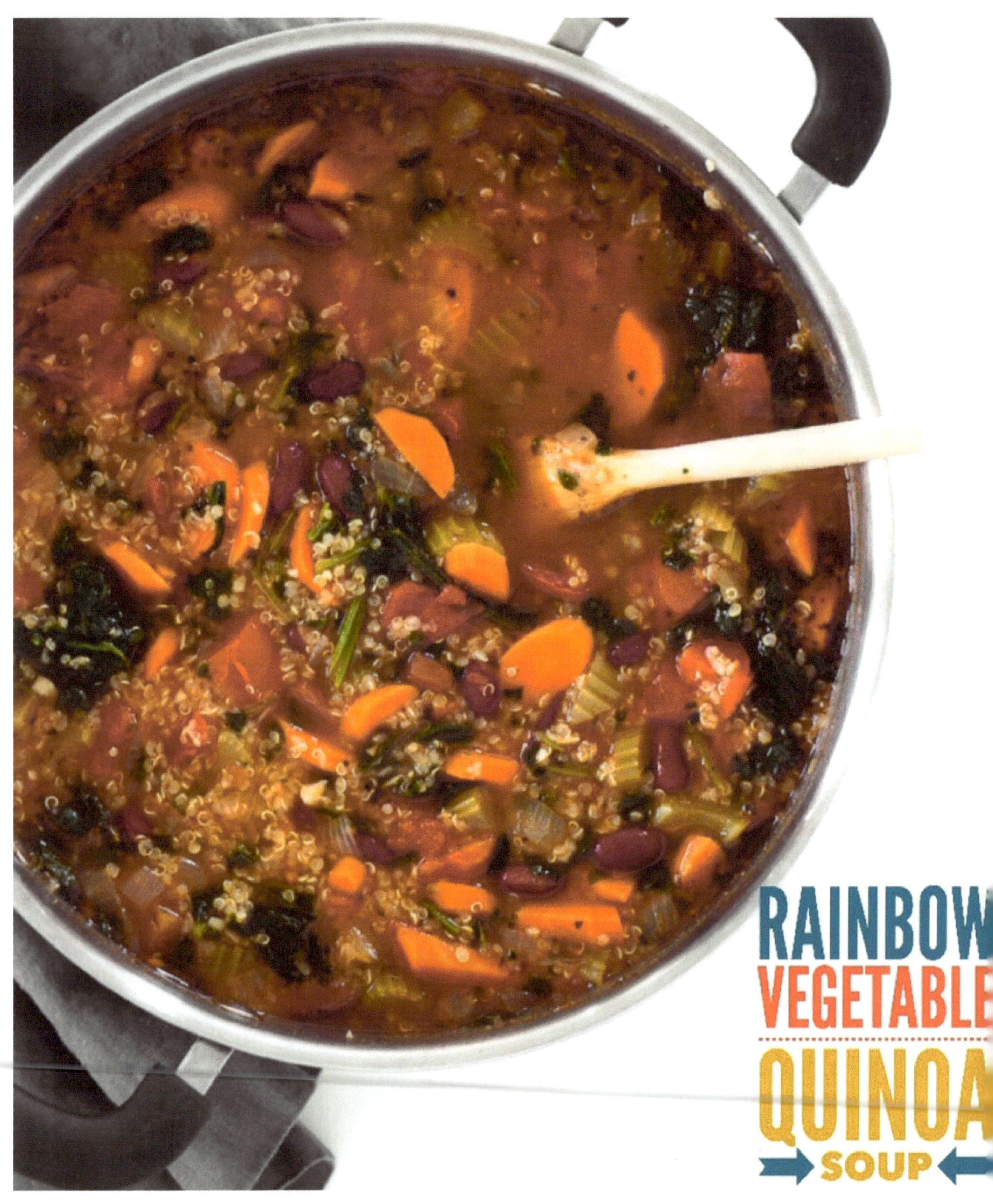
RAINBOW
VEGETABLE
QUINOA
SOUP

As a vegan, protein is everything. And it's not hard to find in a plant-based diet.
Quinoa is loaded with protein, so I throw in my dishes all the time. No protein
deficiency here! You KNOW you're doing something amazing for your body
when you eat the Rainbow Vegetable Quinoa Soup. This soup is beautiful AND gives
us some of the best that the garden has to offer. Choked full of calcium,
beta carotene, protein, fiber and it leaves your wallet full costing under $8 to make.
Pair with Garlic Pita Chips for the perfect bowl

- 2 Tbsp olive oil
- 1 yellow onion diced
- 1 Tbsp minced garlic
- 3 carrots
- 3 celery stalks
- 15oz. can kidney beans
- 15oz. can fire roasted diced tomatoes
- ½ tsp dried basil
- 1 tsp dried oregano
- ½ tsp smoked paprika
- pepper to taste
- 1 Vegetable Bouillon cube
- 1 cup uncooked quinoa
- 4 cups vegetable broth
- 2 cups water
- ¼ lb. frozen spinach

Heat olive oil in a large pot and add your onion and
minced garlic
Sauté over medium heat until the onions are soft and
transparent.
While the garlic and onion are cooking, wash and peel
the carrots, then slice into
¼-inch thick rounds. Wash the celery and slice into ¼-
inch pieces.

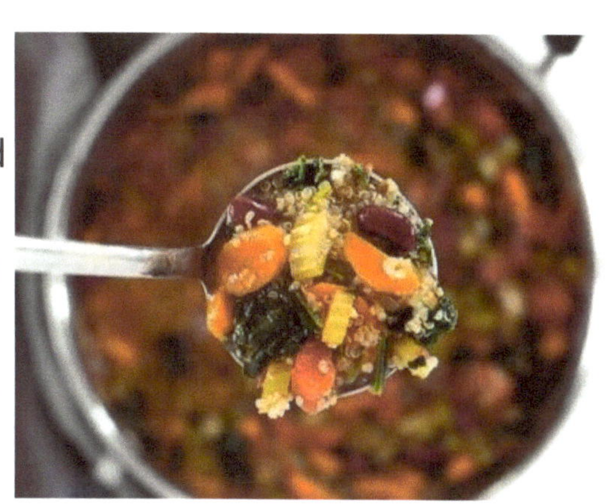

Add the carrots and celery to the pot and continue to sauté until they just begin to soften (about 5 minutes).

While the carrots and celery are cooking, drain and rinse the kidney beans.

Add the quinoa, kidney beans, diced tomatoes (with the juice), basil, oregano, smoked paprika, and pepper to the pot.

Add the vegetable broth, vegetable bouillon cube and water to the pot, place a lid on top and turn the heat up to medium-high.

Allow the pot to come to a boil, then turn the heat down to low and let simmer for 25 minutes.

Stir in ¼ lb. of frozen spinach until heated through. Taste the soup and adjust the seasonings if necessary. Serve hot with Garlic Pita Chips.

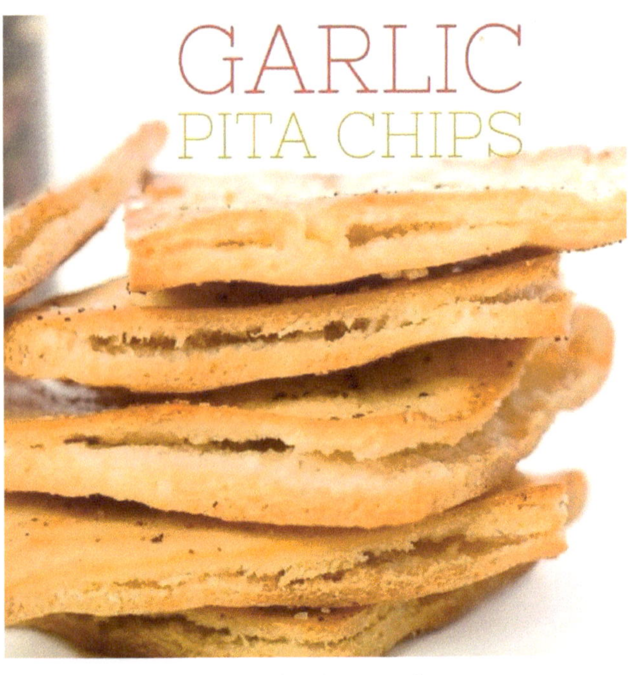

3 pita breads
4 Tbsp olive oil
2 minced cloves or
1 Tbsp of minced garlic
1 tsp of Himalayan pink salt and black pepper

In a bowl mix your olive oil and minced garlic. Cut each of your pita into 8 triangles and place on a baking sheet. Once arranged on sheet brush oil mixture on your 24 pita triangles. Sprinkle with salt and pepper. Place in oven on 350 degrees for 8-10 minutes or until crispy and golden to your liking.

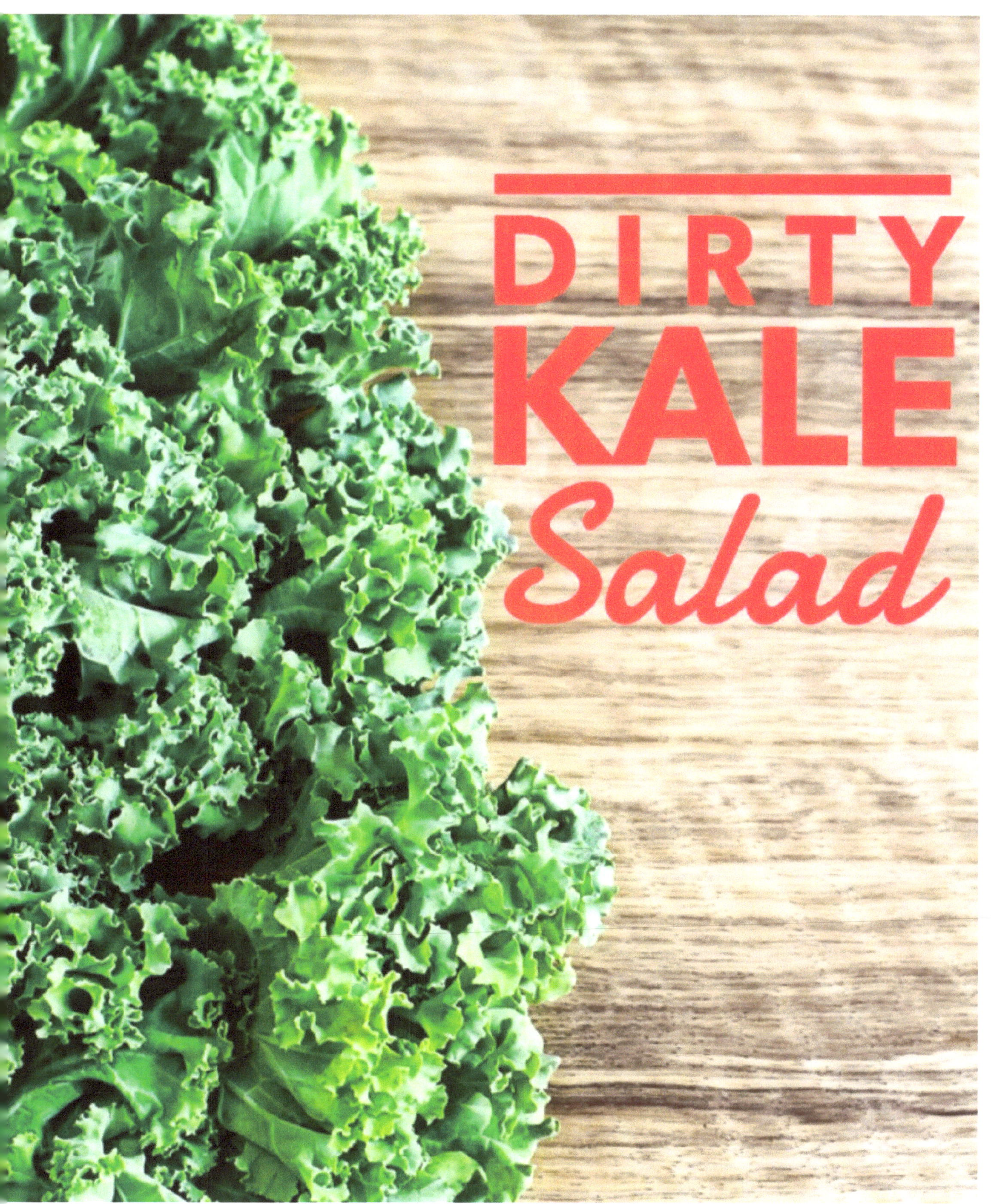

March
DIRTY
KALE
Salad

Spring is in the air! This is a time of freshness and new possibilities. I can't think of a better time to gift you one of my favorite power green salads named
Dirty Kale. The magic of this salad lies in the creamy healthy fat of the avocado. Avocado is one of nature's beauty foods that nourishes our hair, skin
and nails. The good/healthy fat in avocados increases the amount of nutrients our bodies retain from other whole food sources. It is working hard to keep us beautiful from the inside out.
Visit bit.ly/ebdirtykale for a vlog of me making this amazing salad.

1 Bag of Fresh Kale
1 Ripe Avocado
Juice of 1/2 Lemon
2 Tbsp Liquid Aminos
1/2 cup sliced Kalamata Olives
1/2 cup Raisins
2 Tbsp Whole Flaxseeds

Wash hands. Place half the bag of kale in a colander or strainer and massage kale under water as warm as you can take it.
This is a raw dish so aside for making sure the kale is thoroughly cleaned this will soften the kale and ensure the absolute most nutrients are retained and getting into our bodies.
Put softened kale into your salad bowl and now it's time to get dirty. Cut your avocado in half, removing the pit and scooping both sides out into your salad bowl.
Time to put some good energy into this salad by taking both hands and squeezing the avocado thru the kale until it is coated with all the yummy avocado like a creamy dressing.
Rinse your hands and let's add the liquid Aminos, lemon juice (used to keep avocado green), kalamata olives, raisins and flaxseeds. Feel free to get dirty in there again with your hands or use a spoon to fold ingredients together.

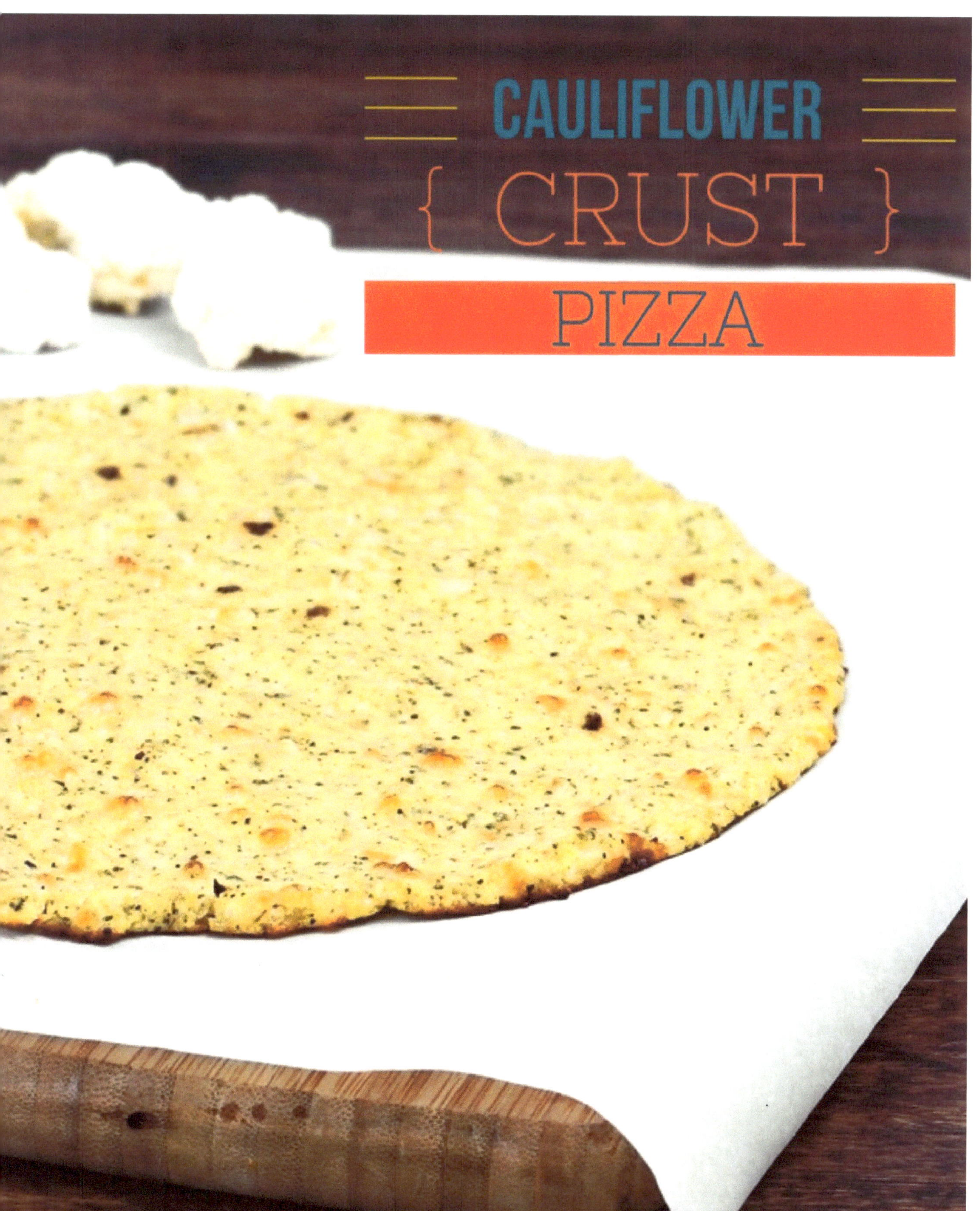
CAULIFLOWER
{ CRUST }
PIZZA

If choosing to include more plant-based foods in your diet leaves you feeling deprived YOU'RE DOING IT WRONG. This recipe is Exhibit A. One of the greatest joys of eating plant based is that I didn't give up any of the amazing foods I enjoyed before…I just made better choices in ingredients. The flavors went nowhere but ALL THE WAY UP! No matter how picky the eater, NO ONE will have a problem with you making Cauliflower Crust Pizza time and time again. AND you are giving them fiber, protein, B vitamins (niacin, riboflavin, folate). Don't let the list of ingredients make you shy away either. A lot of these will become staples in your pantry as you journey into healthy natural living.

- 2 Bags of Frozen Riced Cauliflower
- 2 Tbsp ground flax meal
- 6 tablespoons water
- 1/2 cup corn meal
1/2 cup flour
1 Tbsp Chia seeds
- 1/2 teaspoon salt
- 1/2 teaspoon garlic powder
- 1/2 teaspoon dried oregano Parchment Paper

Preheat oven to 400F
Prepare the frozen cauliflower rice as instructed and let sit in colander to dry away excess moisture (15-20 minutes)
While cauliflower dries make 2 vegan eggs by combining the flax meal and water. Stir and place in fridge uncovered (minimum 7-10 minimum)
Put your Riced Cauliflower in a food processor or blender to make it a little more "mashed". Push down on sides twice more to make sure it all gets attention. (It will look like mashed potatoes)
Place the cauliflower in a large bowl, adding the vegan egg mixture, the almond meal, chia seeds, salt, garlic and dried oregano.

Stir/fold well to mix, then press the mixture onto a parchment-lined pizza pan. Simply use your hands to shape the crust into your desired size, keeping the crust about 1/4-inch thick.

For best results, press the crust together firmly, making sure that there are no thin spots where it might crack.

Bake at for 30 minutes until the top is lightly golden and dry to the touch. Add an additional piece of parchment paper to flip the entire pizza crust over, remove the old piece of parchment paper and bake for an additional 15 minutes for a perfect cauliflower crust.

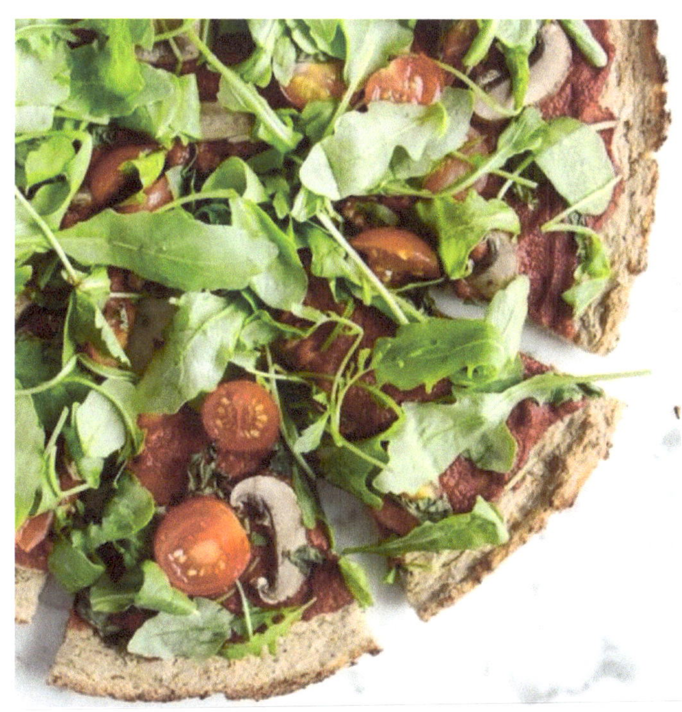

Once the crust is firm and dry, add your organic pizza sauce and any of your favorite pizza toppings. Return to the oven to let everything heat up for 5-10 minutes. My go to toppings are vegan cheese, onions, fresh spinach, kalamata olives, pineapple for my perfect pizza. If you've never had vegan cheese try the Daiya brand at your grocery store.

It is a super cheesy and delicious vegan cheese that melts and stretches. Whatever pizza toppings you choose, I know you will enjoy this vegan recipe! Because of this I recommend doubling or tripling the recipe and freezing the leftover crusts, for an easy pizza night in the future! You and your family will definitely want to make these pizzas again.

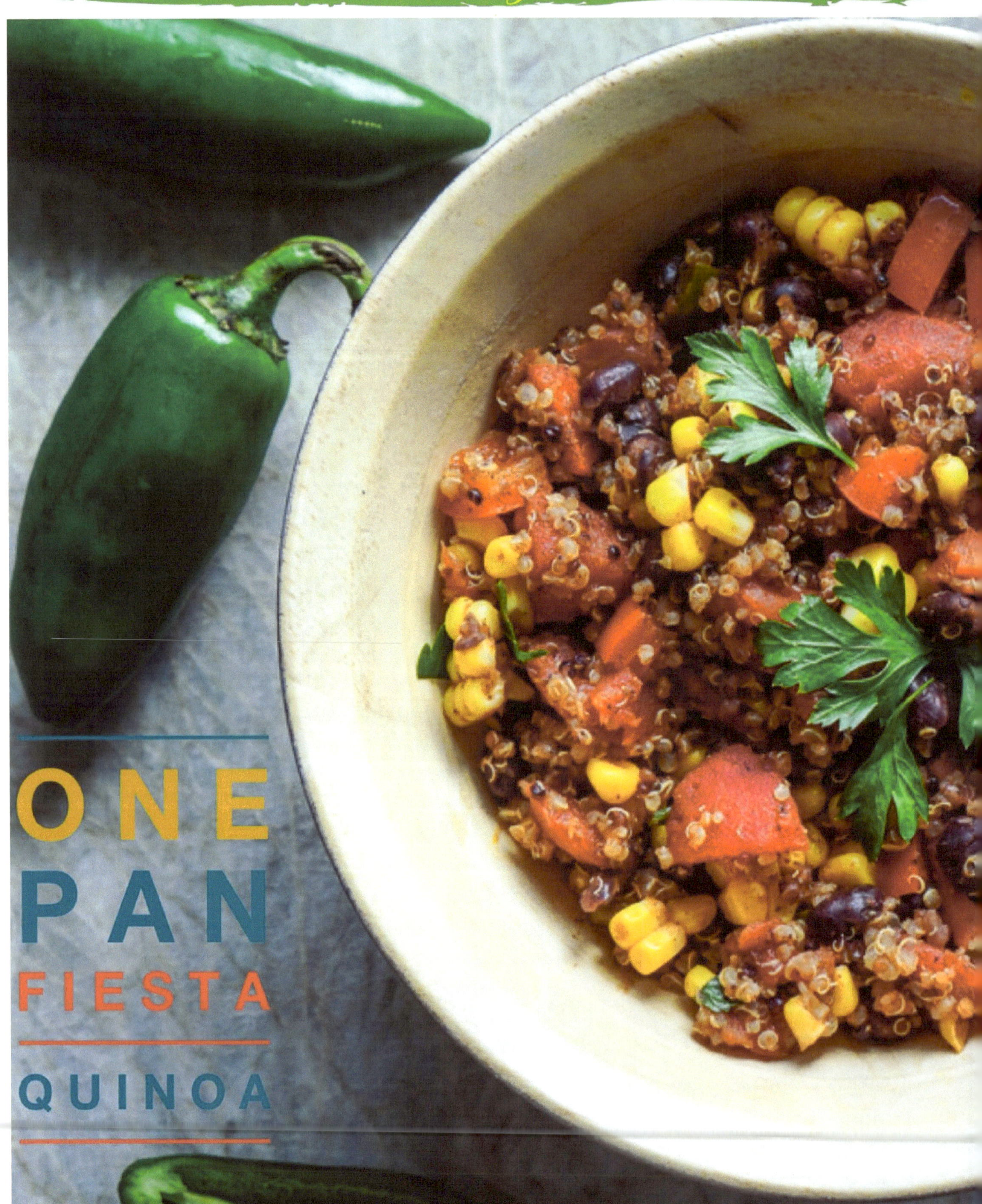

May
ONE
PAN
FIESTA
QUINOA

This is the meal that made me social media famous, HA! The One Pan Fiesta

Quinoa is hands down the quickest, easiest, most nutritious and delicious hot meal you can make for your family. It is loaded full of amazing real food
like the protein from your quinoa and beans, the beautiful healthy fats from
your avocado as well as the antioxidants in your tomatoes and cilantro. Wait until your family gets a load of this! I've come to save you time and make you the hero of tonight's dinner. All you need is 30 minutes and one pan.
I guarantee no one will ask you where's the meat.

- 2 Tbsp olive oil
- 1 tsp minced garlic
- 1 jalapeño minced
- 1 cup dry tri-color quinoa
- 1 cup vegetable broth
- 1 (15-ounce) can black beans, drained and rinsed
- 1 (14.5 oz) can fire-roasted diced tomatoes
- 1 cup frozen corn kernels
- 1 tsp chili powder
- 1/2 tsp cumin
- Himalayan pink salt and freshly ground black pepper, to taste
- 1 avocado, halved, seeded, scoop out and dice
- Juice of 1 lime
- 2 Tbsp chopped fresh cilantro leaves

Heat olive oil in a large skillet over medium high heat. Throw in your minced garlic and jalapeño Cook, stirring frequently for 2 minutes.
Add your dry quinoa, vegetable broth, drained and rinsed beans, tomatoes, corn, chili powder and cumin; season with salt and pepper, to taste.
Stir ingredients together.

Bring to a boil; cover, turn heat down to low until quinoa is cooked, about 20 minutes.
Stir in avocado, lime juice and cilantro.
Have a sneak taste.
Virtually slap ya Mama.
Serve immediately.
Humbly accept your praises.

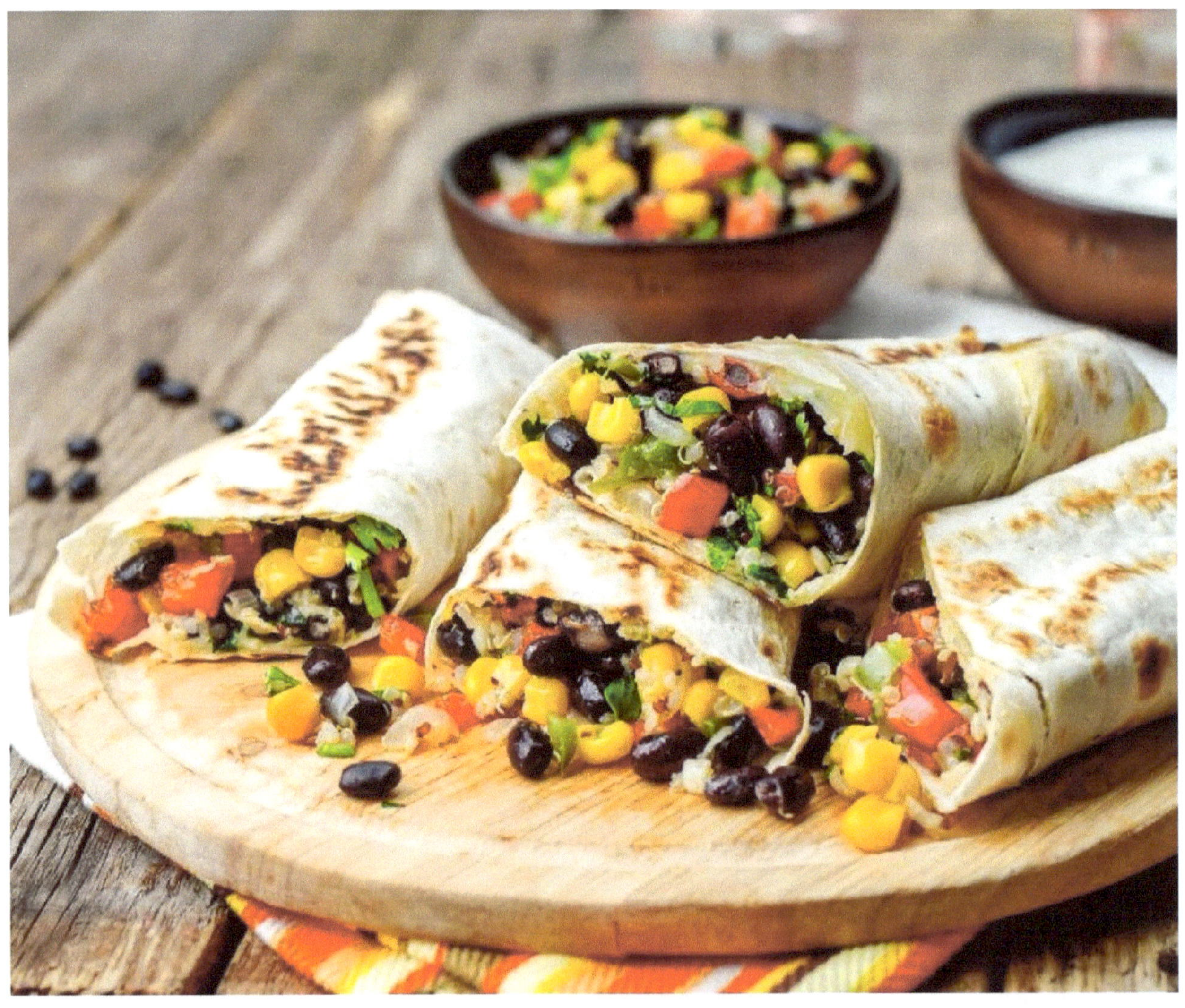

You can't lose with the dish. It stands alone as an awesome main dish or you can make it a side or turn it into wraps.

SPAGHETTI
SQUASH MARINARA

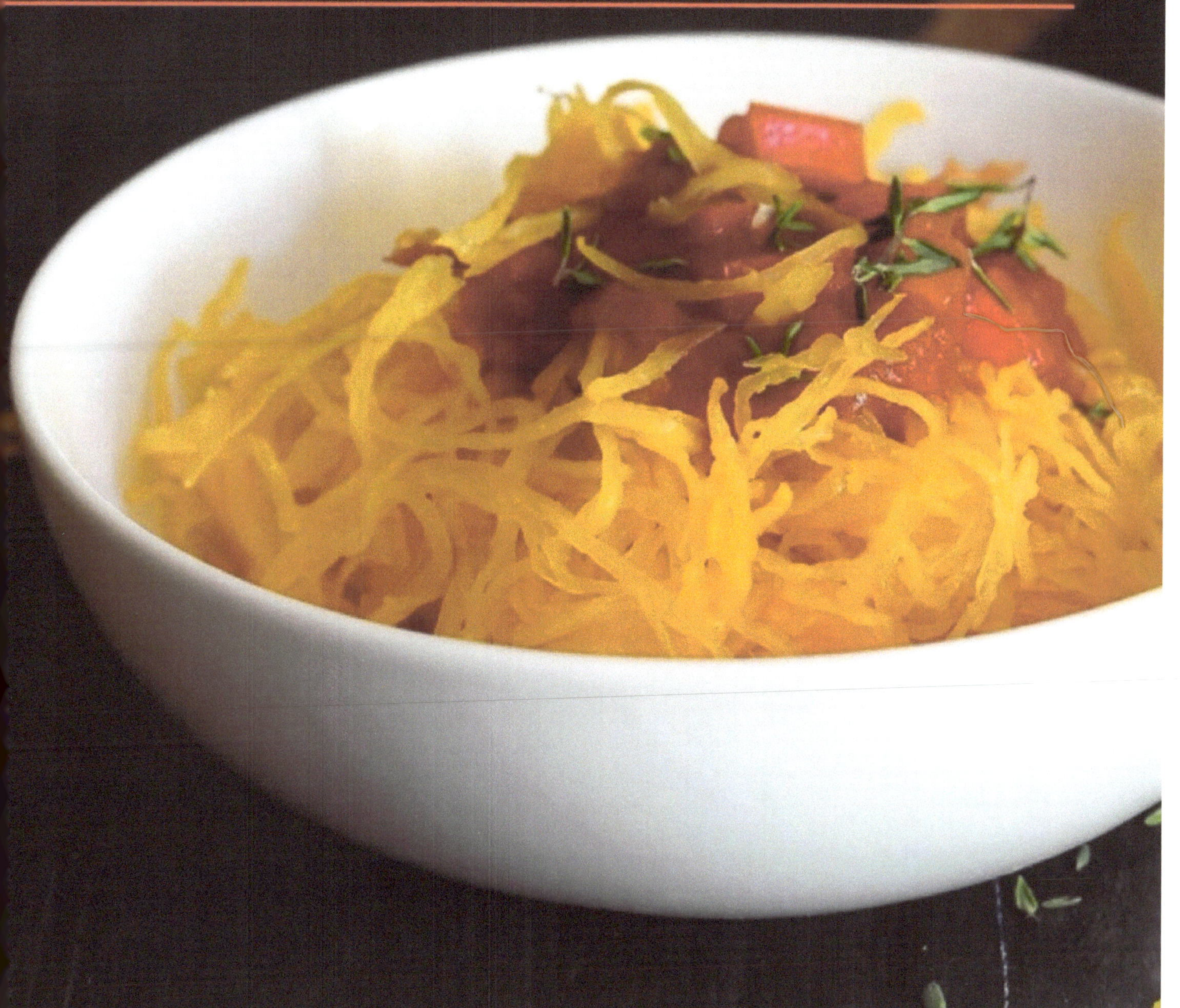

If you love pasta (like me), but aren't so fond of what does to your waist line (like me) then you will love Spaghetti Squash Marinara! I honestly can't tell you the last time we had traditional pasta. My family expects this as their pasta now and soon yours will too.

You can also use meatless meatballs or vegan crumbles for a treat that your family won't even know is vegan.

1 large Spaghetti Squash

1 25.5 oz. jar of organic Marinara Sauce

2 14.5 oz. cans of Fire Roasted Diced Tomatoes

1 10 oz. can Diced Tomatoes in Lime and Cilantro Olive Oil

Himalayan Pink Salt

Pepper

Dried Oregano

1/2 cp Diced Yellow Onion

1 Tbsp Minced Garlic

1/4 cup Fresh Basil

Gardein Meatless Meatballs (Optional)

If you have a pressure cooker you will save yourself some time cooking the squash.

Cut the ends off your spaghetti squash and split them down the middle.

Take a spoon and scoop out the middle and any seeds.

Pour 1 cup of water in your pressure cooker and place the halves on their side facing each other.

Set pressure and timer for 10 minutes.

Once done carefully remove squash from cooker and let cool if needed.

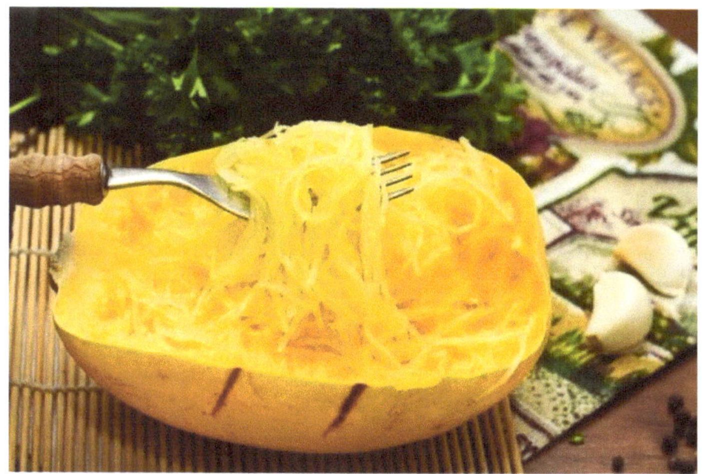

Take a fork and rake long ways of the squash and your spaghetti will appear!
Put it in a dish and drizzle with olive oil and pepper or put marinara on top serving it right out of the squash for a beautiful presentation.

If you don't have a pressure cooker take a glass baking dish and pour 1/2 cp of water in the bottom. Place the halves in the dish upside down. Bake on 450 degrees 30-40 minutes.

Once done follow instructions above to remove your spaghetti. Heat your marinara, fire roasted tomatoes and tomatoes in lime and cilantro in a pot. Add your seasonings and optional meatless meat. Garnish with fresh chopped basil.

Buon Appetito!

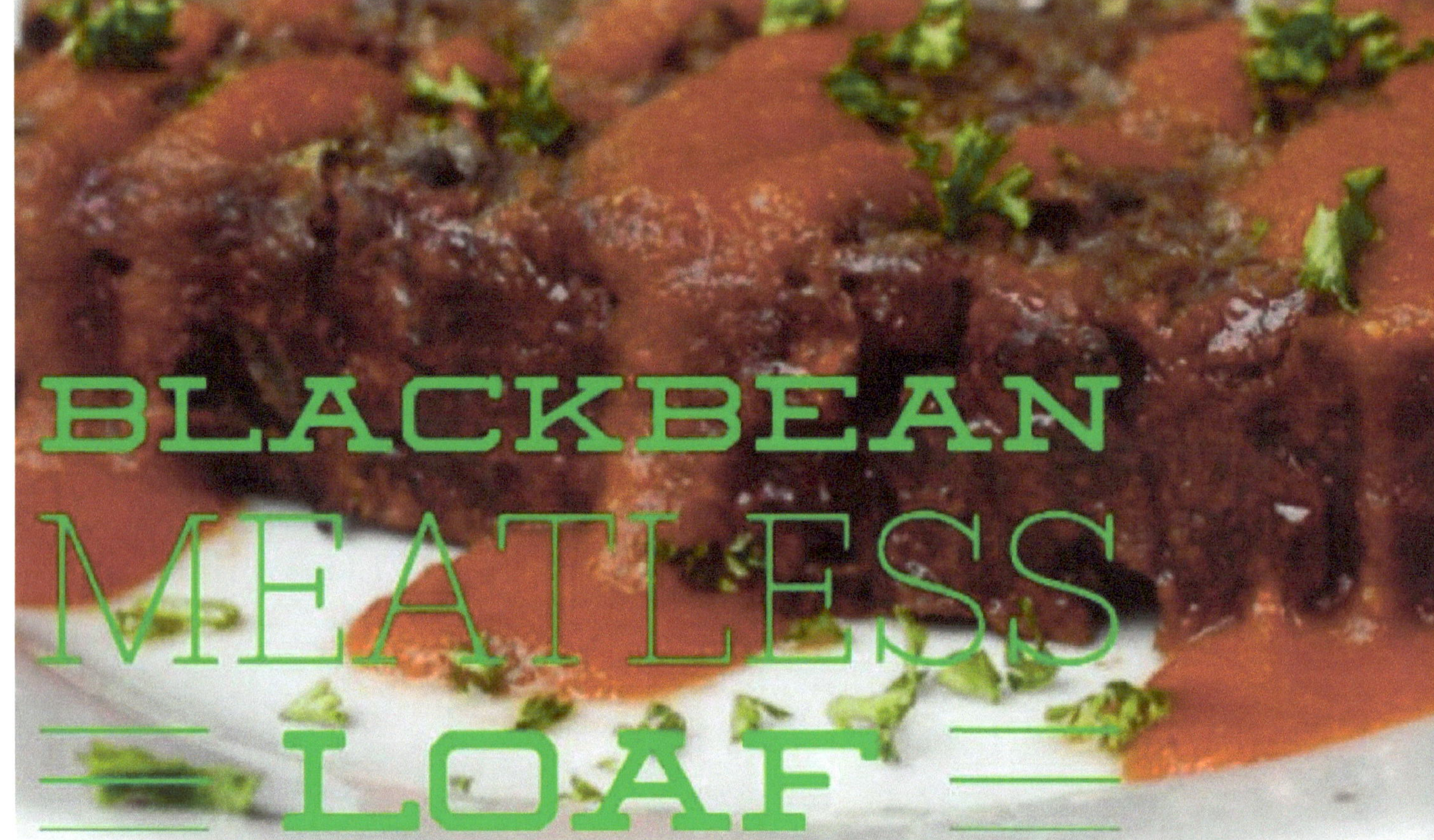

This time of year, we are getting together with family and reminiscing on good times. Some good comfort food would fit in just fine! One of my favorite meals use to be meatloaf, mashed potatoes and green beans so I had to put a plant based spin on it. You will be so surprised how closely the texture and flavors of the Black Bean Meatless Loaf comes to the ol' comfort dish.
Pair it with Roasted Garlic Cauliflower Mash

2 cans of black beans rinsed
1 1/2 cup quick oats
1 red bell pepper chopped
1 carrot chopped or grated
1 yellow onion diced
1/2 Tbsp minced garlic
1 Tbsp Braggs Liquid Aminos
1 tsp Cumin
3 Tbsp organic Ketchup (optional)
3 Tbsp organic Tomato Paste (optional) Black
Pepper Water for sautéing

Pre-heat oven to 350F.
In a medium pan, water sauté the onions until translucent then add the garlic, bell pepper and carrot. Cook for about 5-6 minutes, until softened.

In a large bowl, combine the black beans, oats and all seasonings. Add in the veggies that you sautéed and mash with a potato masher or fork until well combine but not mushy. If it isn't moist enough add water and if too moist add oats until it holds together.

Spoon "meatloaf" into a parchment paper lined loaf pan and spoon ketchup across the top.

Bake for 30 minutes until it has developed a nice crust.
Pour your 50/50 tomato sauce mixture over it and serve with Roasted Garlic Cauliflower Mash.

Cauliflower mash is to mashed potatoes what spaghetti squash is to pasta. Yes they're both vegan, however the first are healthier alternatives. People have challenged me and said these are definitely mashed potatoes...NOPE! Not only is this a healthier substitute, but it's something you can make in advance and actually tastes even tastier after all the flavors have "married" in the fridge.

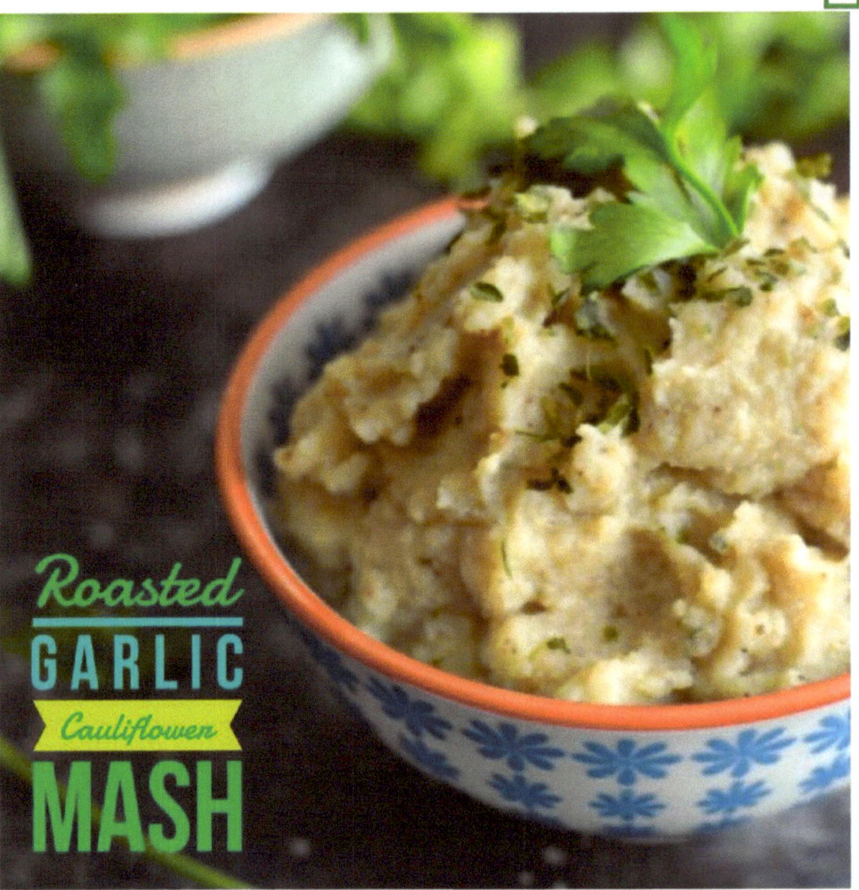

1 head of cauliflower
1 Tbsp of minced garlic
1/3 cup of Almond Milk
Pepper
Himalayan Pink Salt
1/2 Tbsp Parsley
Preheat oven to 375F
Prepare a baking sheet with parchment paper
Clean and slice cauliflower
Place cauliflower on baking sheet, spray with cooking spray & pepper
Roast 40 minutes until edges begin to brown
Remove cauliflower from oven & add to food processor
Add remaining ingredients
Blend 2-3 minutes until a potato like consistency appears
Remove from food processor
Heat on top of stove and serve

August

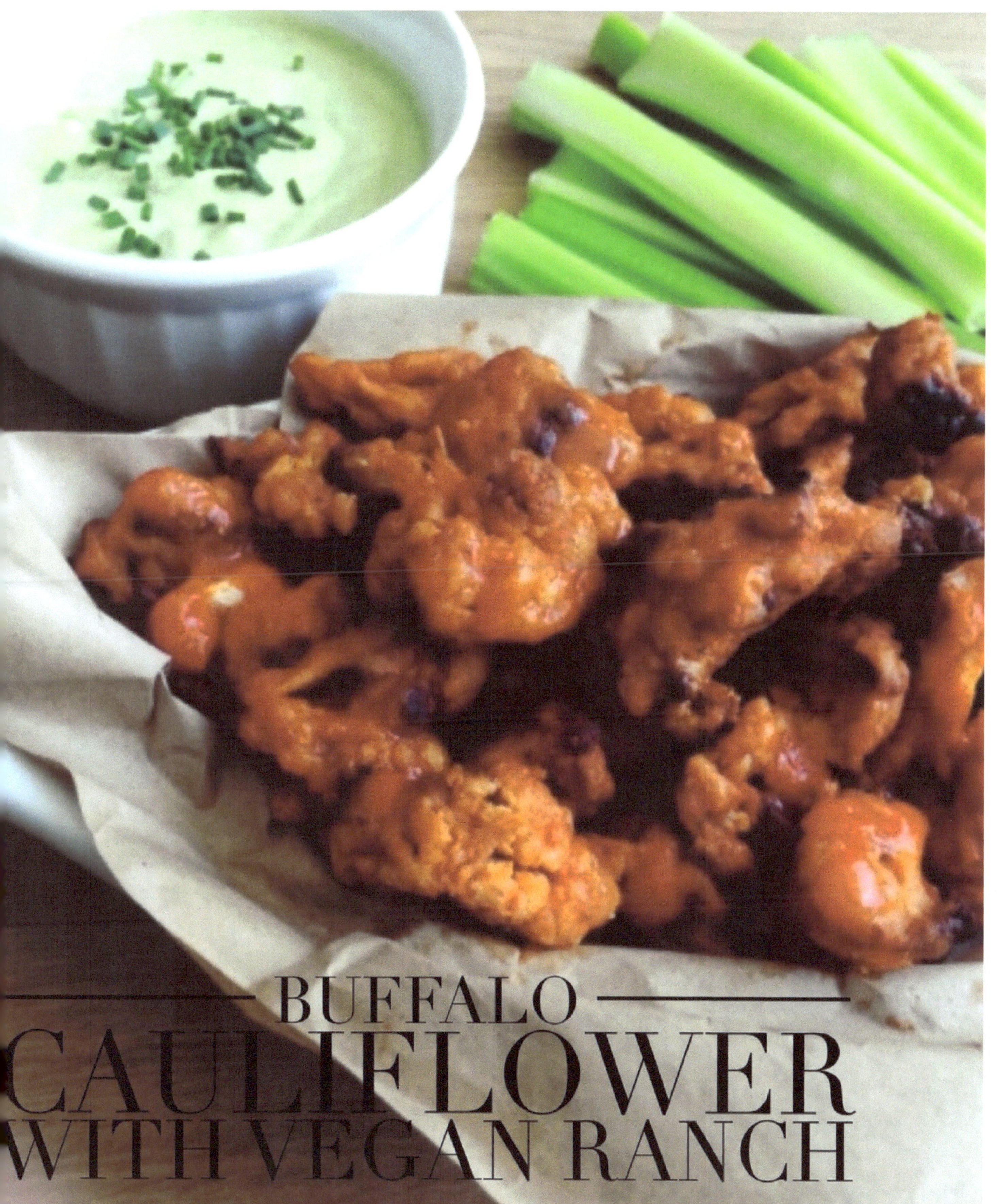
BUFFALO
CAULIFLOWER
WITH VEGAN RANCH

Okay. I have 2 confessions: 1) I thought I would have to give up being a college football fan when I became vegan because what was college game day without a dozen hot lemon pepper chicken wings, mostly flats and something cold to drink?? Turns out I was missing out and now I'm here to help you turn in the prior for these. THEY ARE AMAZING! Like us you will want to have them every weekend. It's not football season with them. And this vegan ranch!... Oh yeah 2) This dish will take you roughly 2 hours from start to finish but stay with me because it's worth it!

1 head of Cauliflower (approx. 4-5 cups of florets)
1/2 cup unsweetened Almond Milk
1/2 cup Water
3/4 cup All-purpose Flour (can sub gluten-free rice flour)
2 tsp Garlic Powder
2 tsp Onion Powder
1 tsp Cumin
1 tsp of Paprika
1/4 tsp Himalayan or Sea Salt
1/4 tsp Ground Pepper
1 Tbsp Earth Balance buttery spread
1 cup Frank's Red Hot Sauce
NOTE: You can substitute 50/50 BBQ and Hot Sauce or use 1 cup of just BBQ sauce for BBQ wings.

Line baking sheet with parchment paper.
Preheat oven to 450 F
NOTE: Parchment paper is essential in preventing the batter from coming off throughout baking! I've tried other methods.
You need parchment paper! Parchment paper and wax paper are NOT the same thing.
Wash and cut cauliflower head into bite sized pieces/florets.
Mix all the ingredients (minus the earth balance and hot sauce, this is added separately!) into a mixing bowl.

Continued

The batter shouldn't be so thick that it doesn't drip, but also not so thin that it
doesn't coat or stick to the cauliflower.
Dip each floret into the mixture and coat evenly. Tap off the excess a couple of times
on the side of the bowl.
Lay florets in an even layer on the parchment lined baking sheet without
overcrowding.
Bake for 25 minutes until golden brown, flipping the florets over half way through to
get all sides golden brown and crispy.
While the cauliflower is baking get your ranch dip and wing sauce
ready. In a small saucepan on low heat melt earth balance and mix in hot sauce.
Remove from the heat just as it starts to melt. Stir together and set aside.
Once the cauliflower is done with its first bake in the batter, remove them from the
oven and put all the baked florets into a mixing bowl with the wing sauce and toss to
coat evenly.
Then spread all the florets in wing sauce out onto the same baking sheet. Bake in the
oven for another 25 minutes, flipping the florets over half way through.
Vegan Ranch
1 cup Vegan Mayonnaise (I recommend Veganaise)
1/8 cup Almond Milk
2 tsp Apple Cider Vinegar
1 tsp Onion Powder
1 tsp Garlic Powder
1/4 tsp Himalayan or Sea salt
1/4 tsp Ground Pepper
1 Tbsp Fresh Dill
1 Tbsp Fresh Parsley
1 Tbsp Fresh Chives
Blend together vegan mayonnaise, almond milk, apple cider vinegar, onion powder,
garlic powder, salt and pepper in a blender. Pour the dip into a jar or serving bowl
and stir in the fresh herbs. Refrigerate before serving. Serve with Celery.

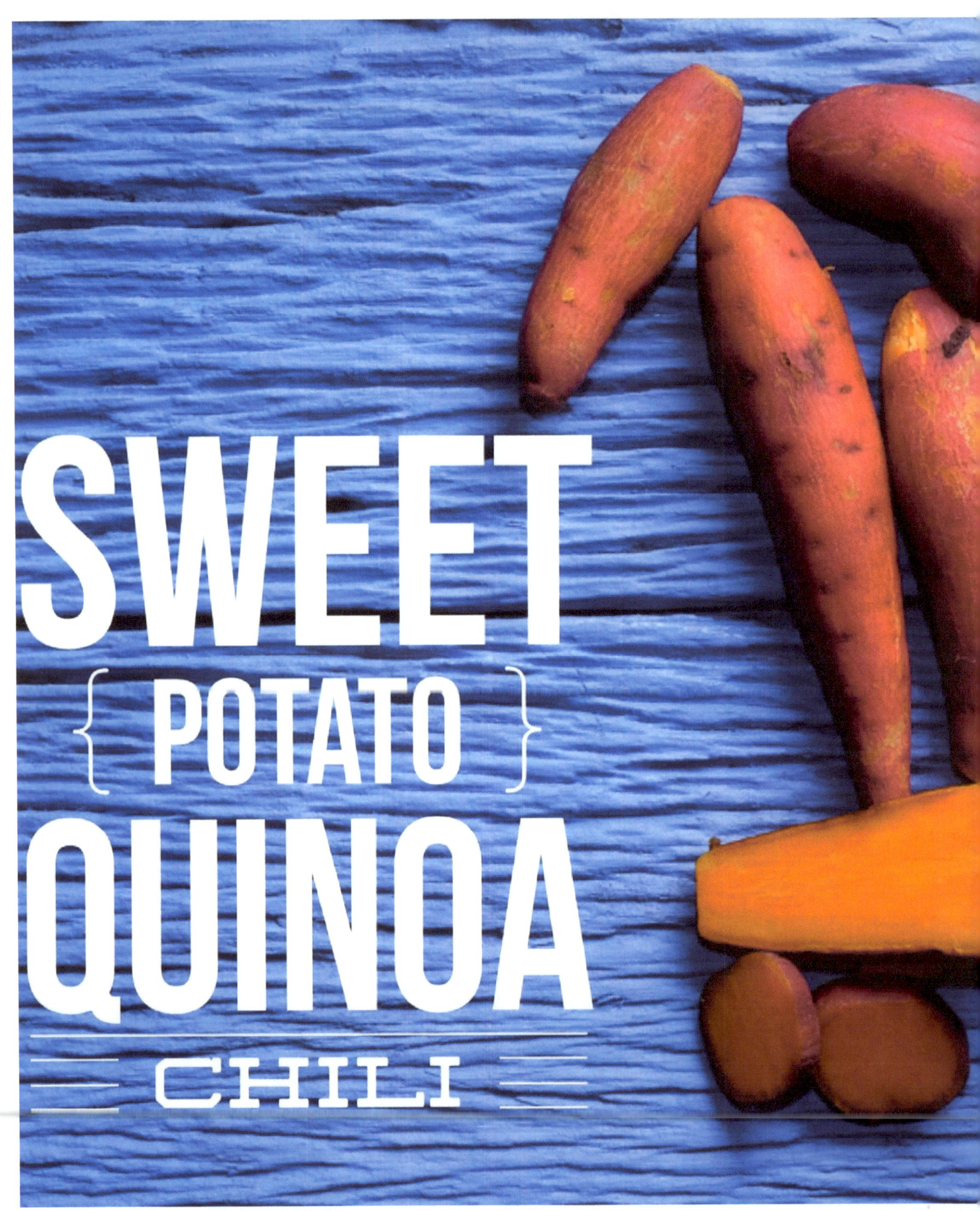
September
SWEET
{ POTATO }
QUINOA
CHILI

Fall is in the air. This is such a beautiful time of year. The leaves are changing, it's time for warmer clothes and OH YEAH, it's sweet potato season!
It's time for hearty soups that load our bodies with the benefits we need to combat the change in the weather. The Sweet Potato Quinoa Chili will fuel your body with tons of protein, beta carotene and anti-inflammatory benefits with vitamins C, A & E.

15 oz. black beans, drained and rinsed

15 oz. kidney beans, drained and rinsed

15 oz. fire roasted diced tomatoes, or 1 1/2 cup diced fresh tomatoes

5 oz. diced tomatoes with lime and cilantro

6 oz. tomato paste

1 large sweet potato peeled and cut into bite sized chunks

1 cup dry tri color quinoa

1 onion diced

1 jalapeño seeded and diced

1 Tbsp. minced garlic cloves

1 Tbsp. olive oil

1 1/2 Tbsp. chili powder

1 Tbsp. Cumin

1 tsp. dried oregano a few dashes

of garlic powder a few dashes of

onion powder

Himalayan pink salt to taste

32 oz. Vegetable broth

Avocado, Fresh Cilantro and Cayenne for garnish (optional but amazing if added)

Continued

In a large pot heat olive oil over medium heat.
Add onions and diced jalapeño, cook until soft and start to turn brown (about 5 – 7 minutes). Add garlic, cook for another minute. Add the tomato paste, chili powder, cumin, oregano, Himalayan pink salt and garlic and onion powders.
Cook for 1 – 2 extra minutes stirring constantly. Add tomatoes, veggie broth, beans and sweet potatoes, stir together.
Add quinoa, bring to a boil, reduce heat to low, cover and cook for 30 minutes, stirring occasionally making sure your chili isn't sticking on the bottom. Add additional broth or water if chili is thicker than you like.
You know it's done when the sweet potatoes are tender.
Top with diced avocado (sprinkled with a little cayenne for color and bit of heat) and cilantro.
Sweet potatoes pack a powerful nutritional punch. They have over 400% of your daily needs for vitamin A in one medium spud, as well as loads of fiber and potassium.
This veggie is an amazing source of beta carotene which gives it its vibrant orange color. The beta carotene is converted to
vitamin A after entering the body. Vitamin A can reduce the risk of developing certain types of cancer and has also been shown to protect against heart disease and asthma. Not to mention that by increasing your intake of plant foods like sweet potatoes you decrease the risk of diabetes, heart disease and obesity while also boosting your energy levels and a healthy complexion.

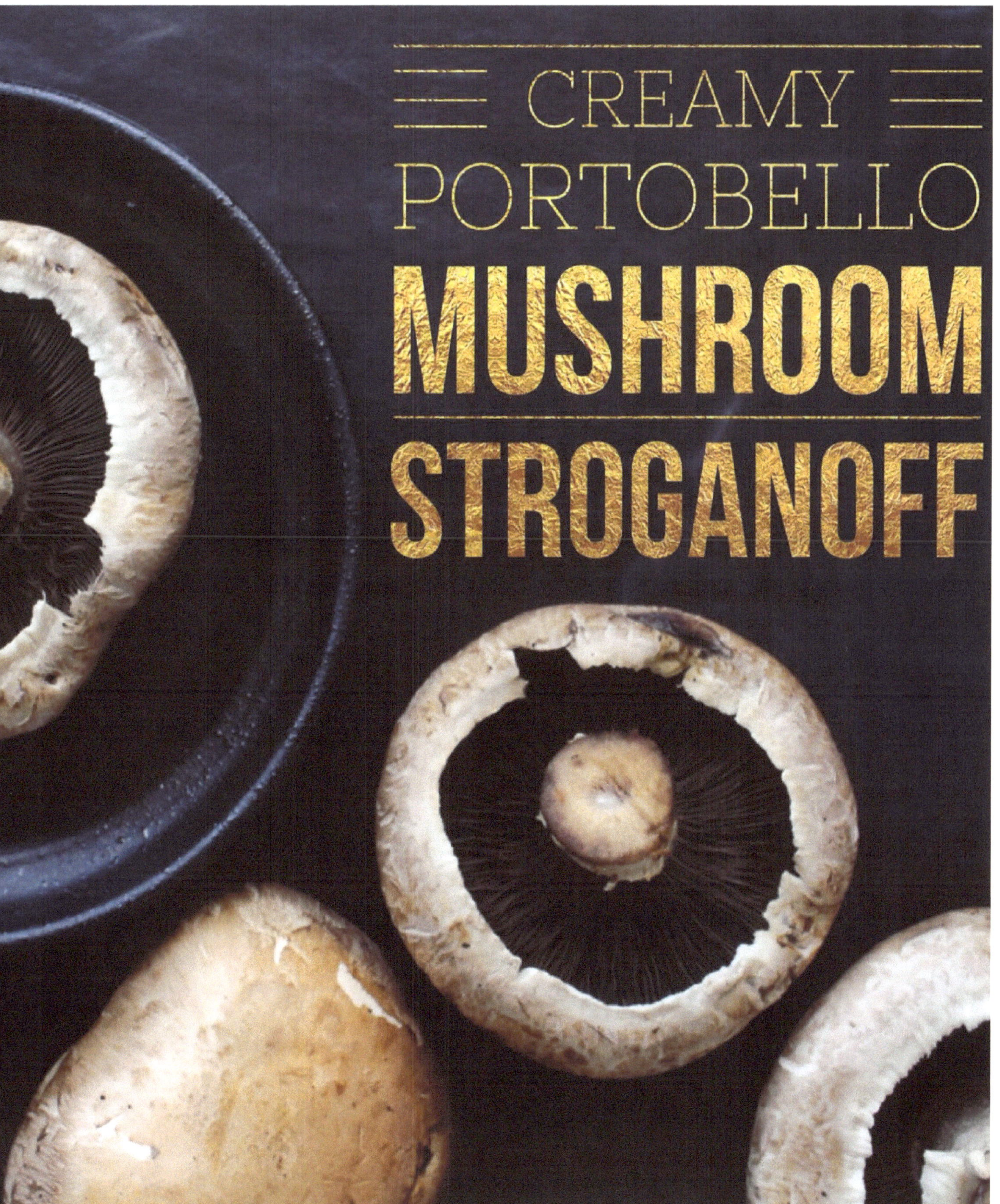
CREAMY
PORTOBELLO
MUSHROOM
STROGANOFF

Oh stroganoff...
Another one of those comfort foods from our childhood that you'd think you would have to give up on a plant-based diet. Not on my watch! The mushrooms are the magic that give the Creamy
Portobello Mushroom Stroganoff its deep flavor and texture that would challenge any carnivore to complain while the cashew cream and herbs top it off with a taste you've never experienced.
And not to mention mushrooms are one of only a few whole foods that naturally contain vitamin D and regulate blood sugar. Dig in!

3 cups Fresh Portobello Mushrooms sliced
1 small Yellow Onion peeled and diced
1/2 Tbsp minced Garlic
1 Tbsp Earth Balance Buttery Spread
2 cups Vegetable Broth
1 cup Raw Cashews
1 Tbsp Fresh Thyme (or 1 tsp dried)
1 Tbsp Fresh Rosemary (or 1 tsp dried)
1 tbsp Fresh Oregano (or 1 tsp dried)

Place cashews and half a cup of water in a blender or food processor and leave to soak. (min 30 minutes - overnight)
In a large pot, sauté the mushrooms, onion and garlic in vegan butter for 3 – 5 minutes, until onions are translucent.
Reduce heat to medium - low and add vegetable broth.
Cover and allow to simmer for 30 minutes.
Blend cashews until smooth and creamy.
Add the cashew cream and herbs to the pot, stirring well to combine.
Allow to simmer for another 20 minutes.
If the stroganoff looks too thick, add a little water.
Season with salt and pepper. Serve over quinoa or spaghetti squash.

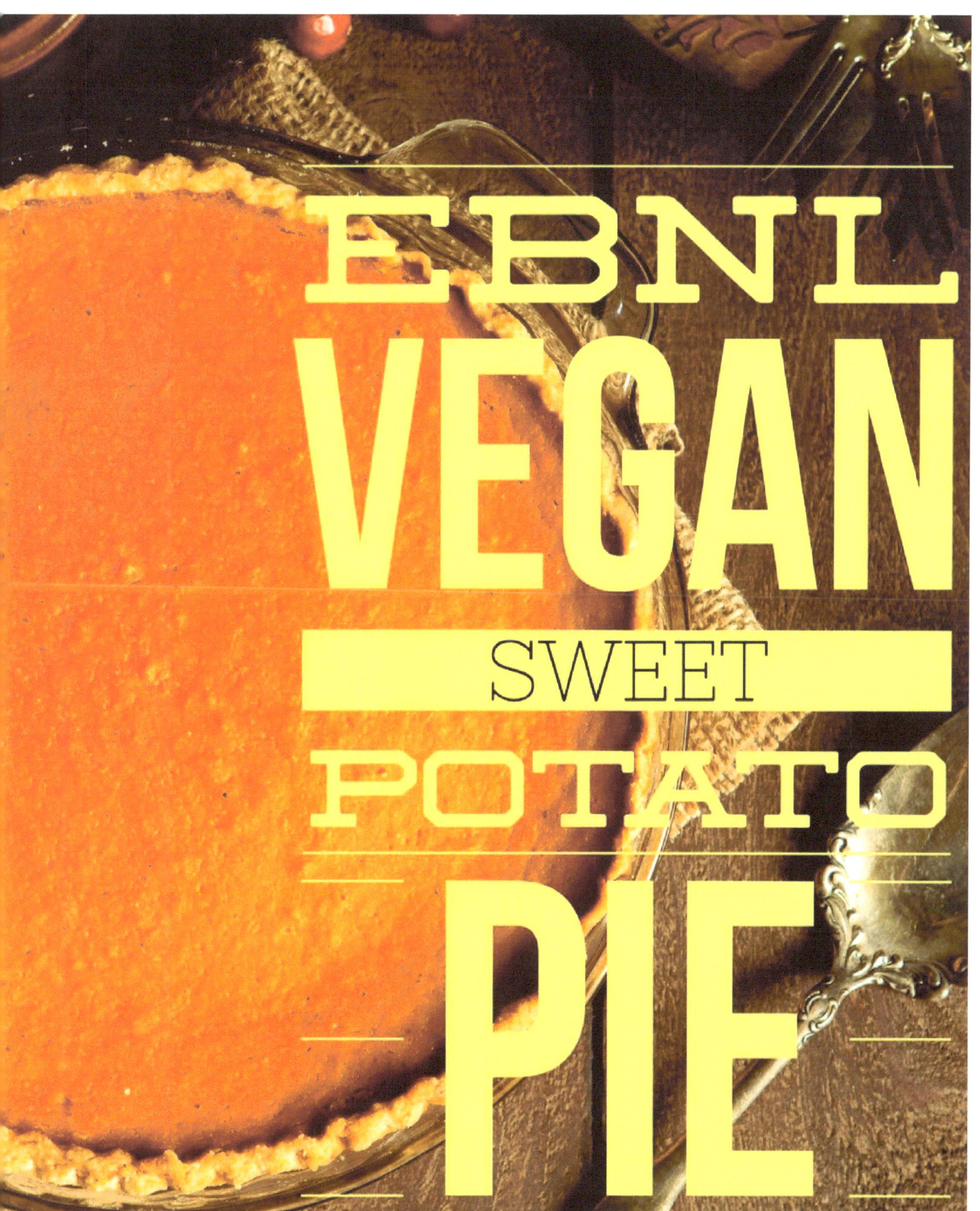
EBNL
VEGAN
SWEET
POTATO
PIE

When I was a kid sweet potato pie tasted
like love. I never grew out of that. When I first became vegan in 2013 the
thought of never having this little piece of heaven again
momentarily had me asking what I was doing to my life. The good
news is that I have a husband who will do everything in his power to make me
happy. This was proven yet again when he began testing
and developing a vegan sweet potato pie recipe during a time that he had no
thoughts of becoming vegan himself. That's love!
This pie has been shared with our family and friends ever since and is
ALWAYS the first pie to be demolished among all the others. We have never
told them it's vegan because that's not important. The important thing is that
it tastes like love.

2 Large Sweet Potatoes
1/2 cup dairy free Butter (Earth Balance)
1 cup Light Brown Sugar
1/2 cup Almond Milk
2 Tbsp Whole Ground Flaxseed Meal
6 Tbsp Water
1/2 tsp Ground Nutmeg
1/2 tsp Ground Cinnamon
1tsp Vanilla Extract
1 9-inch Unbaked Pie Crust
1 to 3 Tbsp Coconut Flour 1
Lemon

Preheat oven to 350

Prepare your vegan egg by mixing 2 Tbsp of ground flaxseed meal with 6 Tbsp of water in a small bowl.
Stir and place in fridge (minimum 5 minutes)
Boil sweet potatoes whole in skin for
40 - 50 minutes or until done. Then submerge potatoes in cold water for 5 minutes and remove skin.

Use a fork or potato masher to break apart in a bowl.
Add softened butter and mix well with mixer.
Stir in sugar, milk, vegan egg, nutmeg, cinnamon and vanilla.
Mix on medium speed until smooth. If mixture is slightly loose, add up to 3 Tbsp of coconut flour 1 Tbsp at a time and beat after each one until you get your perfect consistency prior to baking.

Pour filling into unbaked pie crust.
Place directly on middle rack.
Bake at 350 degrees for 55 - 65 minutes or until toothpick inserted in the center comes out clean. Pie will puff up like a soufflé and then flatten down as it cools.

Let pie cool for 30 minutes then refrigerate for 30 minutes.
This ensure the pie will stand firm once the first piece is cut and plated for the perfect presentation.

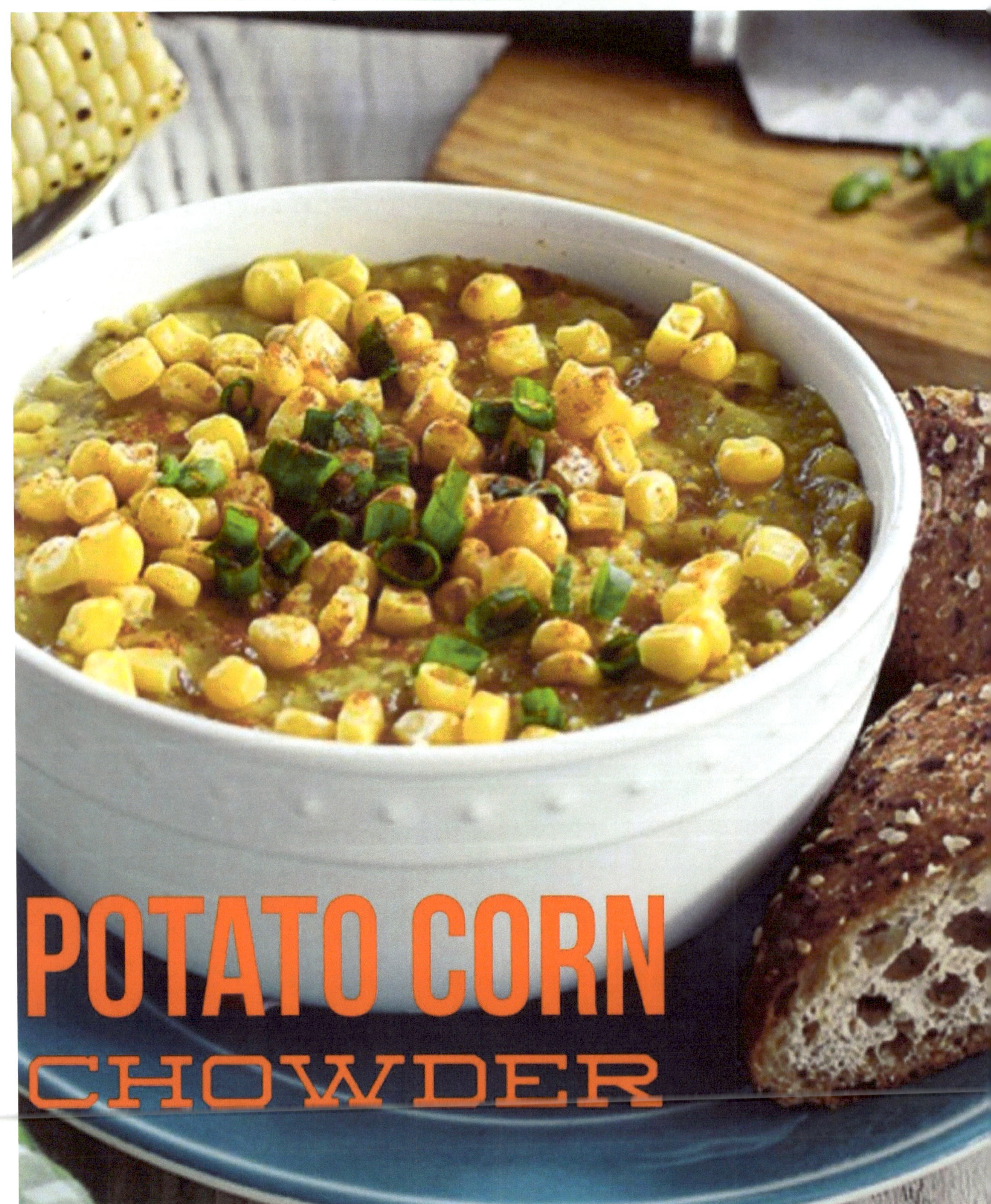

POTATO CORN CHOWDER

Nothing says comfort in the colder months than a nice warm fire and sitting cuddled up with your love while eating a nice big bowl of chunky amazing soup! I can't help you with the first two parts of that perfect evening equation, but the third one I've got you! This will hands down be the best, easiest, creamiest soup recipe you have ever made. And you are getting in a great source of potassium which helps lower and stabilize blood pressure. Remember to keep the skin as that's where the majority of the nutrients lie.

4 Large Potatoes chopped
1 Small Onion chopped
8 Celery Stalks chopped
1/2 Tbsp Minced Garlic
1 1/2 cups Organic Frozen Yellow Corn
1 cup Raw Cashews
1 Tbsp Extra Virgin Olive Oil
1 1/4 tsp Himalayan Pink or Sea Salt
1/4 tsp Celery Seed
7 1/2 cups Water

Over medium high heat add your olive oil, onion, celery and garlic. Sautee until your onions are translucent. Once they are, add your water and potatoes. Cook on medium high until potatoes are tender (12-15 minutes once water gets warm).

After they are tender add corn. Now for the part that makes it creamy! In your blender add 3-4 ladles of your soup including broth and 3 ladles of just broth. Add cashews, celery seeds and salt. Blend until smooth. Add mixture to pot and stir.

And voila! Vegan, creamy, chunky, delicious potato corn chowder. Serve in your favorite soup bowls garnished with smoked paprika and scallions

YOU DID IT!
Congratulations on gifting your body at least 1 meatless meal every month.
Thank you for allowing me into your and your families journey to health natural living.
Share your experience with us by using the hashtags #earthlybodies #ebnlmeatlessmeal #EatYourMedicine #VitaminCAKE
I would love to hear from you on earthlybodies.org or visit me…

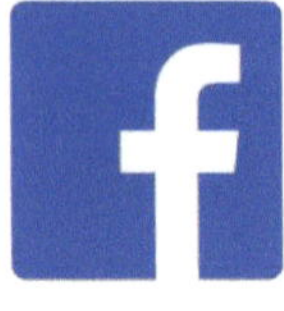
@Earthly Bodies Natural Living

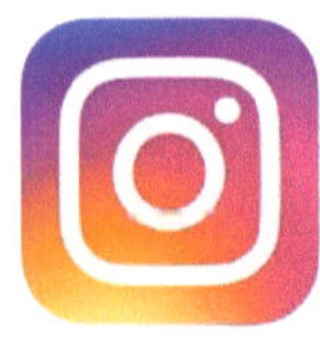
@earthlybodies

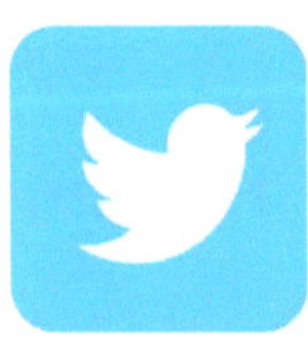
@EarthlyBodies

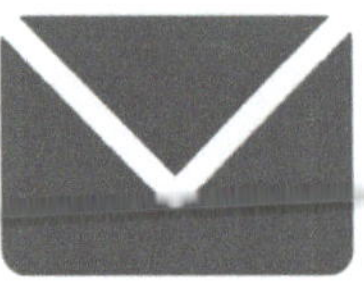
info@earthlybodies.org

NOTES